HOW TO DETECT AND HELP CHILDREN OVERCOME DEPRESSION

Pay Heed Lest You Lose That Child To Depression

by

J. T Mike

Dedication

To Christiana, my sweet sixteen of all seasons, who did not live to read this.

Acknowledgements

To those who attempted or really did assist one way or the other to make this dream a reality, hearty cheers from Yours Truly!

TABLE OF CONTENT

CHAPTER ONE- INTRODUCTION

1.1 What Is Depression?

Depression has been described as a mental illness marked by persistent feelings of sadness, irritability, loss of interest in activities, feelings of hopelessness and worthlessness, and sometimes, thoughts of suicide.

1.2 What Is Childhood Depression?

When 'depression' is a subject matter in any gathering the children are usually excused since it is believed to be an 'adult thing'. Regrettably, the subject matter of this discourse transcends any definite age grand since it is premised on the workings of the mind, albeit may come in various forms hence lack any rigid categorization nor fit into a customized box. Studies have found that first-time depression in children is occurring at younger ages than previously. The research into depression arising during the preschool period (prior to age 6) is relatively new, but empirical data (obtained using narrative and observational methods) have become available that refute traditional developmental theory suggesting that preschool children would be developmentally too immature to experience depression.

The New York Times on February 20, 2019 had in a report titled- 'Teenagers Say Depression and Anxiety Are Major Issues Among Their Peers' confirmed that teens see depression and anxiety as major problem encountered by their peers. Of importance, children having conduct disorder, attention deficit hyperactivity disorder, clinical anxiety, or having cognitive challenge are more prone to sliding into depression. Succinctly, as adults, aged, adolescents battle this, children are not exempted and it interferes with a child's ability to function. It has been observed that preschool depression is more often characterized by age-adjusted manifestations of the typical symptoms of depression than by any other symptom such as aggression.

Appreciating this is the first step in waging a combat against it amongst children who always crave that their mindset can be understood by adults without their appearing stupid! On the flip side, failure to understand this makes a child resort to being unnecessarily cold towards peers or sheer state of temperament, irritable mood or loss of interest in previous pleasurable activities. Recognizing preschool depression can be challenging; common symptoms such as irritability or sadness, when present without other depressive symptoms, are relatively nonspecific markers and cannot be used to differentiate preschool depression from other disorders, though it is established that excessive guilt, extreme fatigue, and diminished cognitive abilities are the most useful markers of preschool depression unlike other early-onset psychiatric disorders. No doubt this is useful to guide the differential diagnosis of early childhood depression. Now, the poser, what can preschool and school-age children be preoccupied with that could lead to depression?

This is usually resultant from a number of biological, societal, psychological, and environmental factors. The prevalence of depression appears to be increasing in successive generations of children, with onset at earlier ages. As will be espoused, low self-esteem, negative social skills, bullying, divorce of parents, child abuse, child labour, not having needs leading to isolation by, peers idleness, negative body image, verbal/physical/sexual abuse, bereavement, setbacks in school, exposure to violence, social isolation, parental conflict, bullying, peer pressure amongst others are factors that can equally cause depression.

1.3 How Common Is Depression In Children?

The National Institute of Mental Health estimates that at least 3.3% of children 13 to 18 years old have had episodes of severe depression. The American Academy of Adolescent Psychiatry estimates this number to be 5%. Biologically, it is said that depression is associated with a deficient level of the neurotransmitter serotonin in the brain, a smaller size of some areas of the brain and increased activity in other parts of the brain. Hence, in treating childhood depression, it is important to address any medical conditions that caused it, counseling, lifestyle adjustments, psychotherapy, and even medication; interpersonal therapy and cognitive behavioral therapy are the major approaches commonly used to treat childhood depression. Timeously addressing childhood depression cannot be termed much ado about nothing, to avert mental problems and disabilities; an apt cliché here being- prevention is better than cure.

1.4 What Causes Depression In Children?

Despite some suggestions of genetic link, depression can occur in people without family histories of depression. Consequently it is important to note that there is no single known cause of depression. Of note, the internet age has made it even more difficult to checkmate childhood depression with e-child abuse, cyber bullying, body shaming, stalking, child pornography and the likes now prevalent. Though trauma, loss of a loved one, difficult times, or any stressful situation may trigger a depressive episode, it results from a combination of influence of multiple genes acting together with biochemical, environmental, and psychological factors.

It has been found that depressive illnesses are disorders of the brain causing parts of the brain responsible for regulating mood, thinking, sleep, appetite, and behavior appear to function abnormally. Hence, Brain-imaging technologies, such as Magnetic Resonance Imaging (MRI), have confirmed that the brains of people who have depression have modifications when compared to people not battling depression. Regrettably, these images do not reveal why the depression occurred.

Whereas the recovery rate from a single episode of major depression in children and adolescents is quite high, reoccurrence cannot be ruled out. Early treatment of childhood depression can reduce its duration and severity and associated functional impairment. As in adults, depression in children can be caused by any combination of factors that relate to physical health, life events, family history, environment, genetic vulnerability and biochemical disturbance. Depression is not a passing mood, nor is it a condition that will go away without proper treatment. It has been found that in childhood, both sex are at equal risk for depressive disorders, but during adolescence, girls are twice as likely as boys to develop depression.

1.5 Depressive Symptoms In Children

Infants and preschoolers do not have the ability to express feelings of sadness in apt language. Therefore, depressive symptoms must be inferred from overt behavior. Of note, when examining disorders amongst children such as depression parents/guardians often fail to spontaneously report symptoms (eg- changes in play, social interest or sleep) or may unwittingly accommodate these changes as being normal.

Symptoms of major depressive disorder common to adults, children and adolescents are:

-Persistent feelings of sadness, anxiety, or feeling "empty"

-Feelings of hopelessness or pessimism

-Feelings of guilt, worthlessness, or helplessness

-Loss of interest or pleasure in hobbies and activities that were once enjoyable

-Decreased energy, fatigue, or feeling "slowed down"

-Difficulty concentrating, remembering, or making decisions

-Insomnia, early-morning awakening, or oversleeping

-Appetite and/or weight loss or overeating and weight gain

-Thoughts of death or suicide; suicide attempts

-Restlessness, irritability

-Persistent physical symptoms that do not respond to treatment, such as headaches, digestive disorders, and chronic pain

Children with depression may also experience the classic symptoms but may exhibit other symptoms as well, including-

- Impaired performance of schoolwork
- Persistent boredom
- Quickness to anger
- Frequent physical complaints, like headaches and stomachaches
- More risk-taking behaviors and/or showing less concern for their own safety.
- Crying more often
- Increased sensitivity to happenings in their environment
- More irritable mood than usual
- Weight loss, headaches or pains
- Disorder in eating pattern or sleeping pattern
- Social withdrawal
- Feeling of dejectedness or disinterest
- Overly pessimistic
- Engaging in self inflicted hurt or other potentially harmful behavior
- Nervousness
- Frequent vague, nonspecific physical complaints
- Loss of interest in school or poor performance in school
- Talk of or efforts to run away from home
- Outbursts of shouting, complaining, unexplained irritability, or crying
- Being bored and disinterest in playing with friends

- Social isolation, poor communication
- Fear of death
- Extreme sensitivity to rejection or failure
- Increased irritability, anger, or hostility
- Reckless behavior
- Older children who are depressed may misuse drugs or alcohol.

Some of the above will be briefly discussed, viz:

-Depressed Mood : Depressed mood, such as feeling low, down, sad, or blue much of the time, is a key symptom of depression which should not be overlooked. This could be evidenced by perceiving others as antagonistic or uncaring, brooding about real or potentially unpleasant circumstances, angry outbursts, maintaining a gloomy hopeless outlook, amongst others. Children find it difficult to get over this unlike adolescents who may decide to get involved in social interactions.

Restlessness or sluggishness: Hand-wringing, pacing, fidgeting, reduced vigour for activities and slow body movements are evident in this category

Fatigue: Childhood depression could lead to a child develop trouble starting or completing tasks.

Feelings of guilt: The feeling of worthlessness and inferiority complex exemplifies this.

Change in appetite or weight: In children, a decrease in appetite may manifest.

Sleep disorder: Childhood depression could lead to a child having trouble getting to sleep, wake in the middle of the night and have trouble getting back to sleep, or wake too early and be unable to get back to sleep or even an outright reversal of sleep cycles whereby they sleep during the day and stay awake at night.

Diminished interest or pleasure: Childhood depression could lead to a child not feeling pleasure doing the things he or she used to enjoy; the medical term for this is- anhedonia.

Impaired concentration: Childhood depression could lead to a child to process information more slowly or become indecisive and unable to take action.

1.6 Difference Between Childhood Depression And Depression Amongst Adult

The diagnostic criteria and key defining features of major depressive disorder in children and adolescents are the same as they are for adults and it has been confirmed that childhood depression tends to be a predictor of severe illness in adulthood. Admittedly, there are some similarities between childhood depression and adult depression to adult depression, particularly as it relates to symptoms, but there are differences between the two, some of which are hereunder set out-

- For younger children, there is a peculiar expression of symptoms which is a fruit of childhood innocence unlike the way an adult expresses depressive disorders

- Another noticeable difference is that children have higher rates of internalization; thus it is more difficult in identifying symptoms of childhood depression. Because these signs may be viewed as normal mood swings typical of children as they move through developmental stages, it may be difficult to accurately diagnose a young person with depression. For instance, diagnosis of the disorder may be more difficult in youth for several reasons, equally, a child with depression may pretend to be sick, refuse to go to school, cling to a parent, sulk, get into trouble at school, be negative and irritable, and feel misunderstood.

- One major cause of this difference is that many of the neurobiological effects in the brain of children with depression are not fully developed until adulthood. Therefore, in a neurological sense, children and adolescents express depression differently.

- Before puberty, boys and girls are equally likely to develop depressive disorders. By age 15, however, girls are twice as likely as boys to have experienced a major depressive episode.

- Depression in adolescence comes at a time of great personal change; boys and girls are forming identities distinct from those of their parents, grappling with gender issues and emerging sexuality, and making independent decisions for the first time in their lives. Depression in adolescence frequently co-occurs with other disorders such as anxiety, disruptive behavior, eating disorders, or substance abuse. It can also lead to increased risk for suicide.

CHAPTER TWO- TREATMENT AND PREVENTION OF CHILDHOOD DEPRESSION

2.1 Treatment of Childhood Depression

Depression is a treatable disorder, even in the most severe cases. Once diagnosed, a person with depression can be treated with a number of methods. It is advisable as a primary step to visit a certified health care provider since some other medical conditions can cause symptoms as found in cases of depression. A certified health care provider such as a doctor can rule out these possibilities by conducting a physical examination, interview, and lab tests. If a certified health care provider can eliminate a medical condition as a cause, a psychological evaluation can be conducted to determine the appropriate health professional to handle such person. The certified health care provider should discuss any family history of depression, and get a complete history of symptoms—when they started, how long they have lasted, their severity, and whether they have occurred before and if so, how they were treated.

Some notable treatment techniques effective in treating children diagnosed with depression are:

-Talk therapy

-Cognitive therapy

-Behavioral therapy

-Interpersonal therapy

-Psychotherapy

- Psychodynamic therapy

Further, Children can get depressed, and disorders ranging from major depression to bipolar disorder. Psychotherapy is often a highly effective form of treatment, and depending on the severity of the case, medication may also be prescribed though in rare cases. This could be cognitive-behavioral therapy (CBT) and interpersonal therapy (IPT). Psychotherapy is often used as an initial treatment for milder forms of depression. It may be accompanied by an early follow-up appointment may help to establish the persistence of depression before a decision is made to try antidepressant medications.

The health care provider consulted to assess a child for depression will likely perform or refer for a thorough medical interview and physical examination as part of assigning the correct diagnosis. This diagnosis can take the form of routine laboratory tests during the initial assessment to rule out other causes of symptoms; an X-ray, scan, or other imaging study. Psychotherapy and medications are common treatment options. On the other hand, talk therapies help patients gain insight into and resolve their problems through verbal exchange with the therapist, sometimes combined with homework assignments between sessions. Psychodynamic therapy focus on resolving the patient's conflicted feelings.

Since children often find it difficult to explain how they're feeling hence, depression can stop kids enjoying the things they normally like doing, or taking part in their usual activities. Treatment options may include alleviating any medical condition that causes or worsens depression. Treatment for children with depression may last for six months to a year depending on the severity of the depression.

In summary, as captured above, treatment may include supportive therapy, like lifestyle and behavioral changes, psychotherapy ("talk therapy" - mental health counseling that entails working with a trained therapist to overcome depression for example through massage of infants or singing for babies), interpersonal therapy(to help the child develop more effective skills for coping with their emotions), cognitive behavioural therapy (this assist the child change his or her way of thinking about certain issues) complementary treatments, and possibly medications (selective serotonin reuptake inhibitor are well known in this regard; and if this fail, dietary supplements like vitamin C and B complex vitamins or other antidepressant medication may be prescribed viz- bupropion (Wellbutrin), venlafaxine (Effexor), duloxetine (Cymbalta), desvenlafaxine(Pristiq), or levomilnacipran (Fetzima))for moderate to severe depression.

However some children will experience some reactions to antidepressant medications, such as insomnia, blurred vision, constipation, and dizziness. Hence, medication as a first-line course of treatment is appropriate for children and adolescents with severe symptoms of depression that would prevent effective psychotherapy, those who are unable to undergo psychotherapy, those with psychosis, and those with chronic or recurrent episodes. Following remission of symptoms, continuation of treatment with medication and/or psychotherapy for at least several months may be desireable to avert relapse and recurrence of depression.

Thus, it is advised that where antidepressants are employed though not advisable in the treatment of depression for children or adolescents, the clinician should monitor closely for adverse symptoms.

2.2 What Are The Treatment Options?

Depression is increasing in successive generations of children, with onset at earlier ages. Of note, finding a lasting remedy to depression and its treatment for children share similarities to the procedure for adults; though with some differences. For instance, with respect to children, antidepressants if ever recommended by medical personnel need to be used with caution to avert hyperactive behavior in children with bipolar disorder. Of note, bipolar disorder is more prevalent in adolescents than in children of tender age. However, bipolar disorder in children can be more severe than in adolescents and may occur with, or be hidden by attention deficit Hyperactivity Disorder (ADHD), Obsessive-Compulsive Disorder (OCD), or Conduct Disorder (CD).

It is worthy to note that a combination of psychotherapy and medication is most effective at treating depression; thought, medications are appropriate where there are other coexisting illnesses. Nonetheless, Health Care Providers may suggest psychotherapy first, and consider antidepressant medicine as an additional option where there is no major improvement in the child's state of mind. In summary you have questions or concerns, discuss them with your health care provider. Additionally, if a child is placed on these medications, it is still very important to continue to follow closely with the Health Care Providers and ask questions since ultimately, there is no general prescription due to differences in children's mental state.

Studies show that the antidepressant Prozac is effective in treating depression in children and teens. The drug is officially recognized by the FDA for treatment of children ages 8 to 18 with depression. Remarkably, there is very little scientific evidence aiding the treatment of early childhood depression. Hence, clinicians are left in dilemma attempting to ameliorate the symptoms and suffering of these innocent souls. In addressing mood disorders, focus is placed on a newly developed key module enhancing emotion development.

Early psychotherapeutic and behavioral approaches have shown promise in the treatment of disruptive disorders in early childhood. Notable health care providers handling depression amongst preschool and school age children have adopted psychotherapies known to be effective in adult and adolescent depression; in particular cognitive-behavioral therapy (CBT) and interpersonal psychotherapy, have been adapted for use in school-age children.

PCIT-ED on the other hand is a manualized 14-session psychotherapeutic treatment. Herein, a microphone and earbud are used during interactions with the child in session thereby allowing the therapist, who observes through a one-way mirror, to provide in vivo coaching. Early intervention targeting developmental skills during the preschool period is equally important in treating a good number of early childhood mental disorders. High vigilance on the part of parents and clinician for the possibility of side effects should be considered since children react differently to treatments of childhood depression.

2.3 What You Can Do To Help Children Overcome Depression

-Listen openly, without judgement

-Revisit the problem

-Keep a focus on normal routines and activities of your child both online and offline

-Get social with your child

- Let your child know that it's OK to ask for help

-Try doing something fun

-Talk about what's going on and how they're feeling

2.4 Seeking Professional Support

Since depression affects the way the child thinks, see himself/herself , The Health Care Providers to consider in diagnosis of clinical depression are-

-Mental Health Counselors

-Pediatricians

-Emergency Room Doctors

-Psychiatrists

-Psychologists

-Psychiatric Nurses

-Nurse Practitioners

-Physician Assistants

2.5 Seeking Assistance From Health Care Providers In Treating Childhood Depression

Depression is a serious illness, but it is a treatable one. Evaluation should include a complete medical assessment to rule out underlying medical causes. Clinicians must rely heavily on parental history, evaluation of parent-child interactions and play interviews by appropriately trained professionals. The longer it goes on, the more likely childhood depression disrupts a child's life and turn into a long-term problem. In the United States, the prevalence of major depressive disorder is approximately 1 percent of preschoolers, 2 percent of school-aged children and 5 to 8 percent of adolescents. The prevalence of depression appears to be increasing in successive generations of children, with onset at earlier ages. The gender ratio has been observed to be equivalent in prepubertal children and increases to a 2:1 female-to-male ratio in adolescents. For instance, it is reported that in the United States, the prevalence of major depressive disorder is approximately 1 percent of preschoolers, 2 percent of school-aged children and 5 to 8 percent of adolescents.

2.6 Can Depression In Children Be Prevented?

Childhood Depression is manifested by a combination of symptoms that interfere with the ability to work, study, sleep, eat, and enjoy once pleasurable activities. Children with a family history of depression are at greater risk of experiencing depression themselves. Children who have parents that suffer from depression tend to develop their first episode of depression earlier than children whose parents do not. Children from chaotic or conflicted families, or children and teens who abuse substances like alcohol and drugs, are also at greater risk of depression. Of note, ultimately loved ones have a major role in improving a child's good mental health. a family history of depression and exposure to stressful life events are the most robust risk factors for depression. Moreso, behaviors that tend to foster attachment of parents with children involve consistent love, care and listening.

The preventive measures includes:

-Addressing risk factors

-Strengthening other protective factors

-Using an appropriate approach for the child's developmental level

CHAPTER THREE- SIMILARITIES BETWEEN CHILDHOOD DEPRESSION AND SIMILAR DISORDERS

3.1 Classes of Depressive Disorders

As a starting point, a distinction is to be drawn between mania and lows. Whereas persistent depressive disorder involves long-term (two years or longer) but the less severe one entails symptoms that keep an individual from functioning well or from feeling good. The following depressive disorders have been identified to influence the mood, mannerisms, functioning and adjustment of young people:

- Major depressive disorder (unipolar depression)

- Persistent depressive disorder (formerly called dysthymic disorder, this is a chronic, mild depression)

- Disruptive mood dysregulation disorder (chronic, severe irritability)

- Premenstrual dysphoric disorder (depressed mood, irritability and anxiety during the pre-menstrual period).

- Bipolar disorders (manic-depression) also have a depressive component.

Admittedly, some forms of depressive disorder exhibit slightly different characteristics than those described above, or they may develop under unique circumstances such as depression with psychotic features, which occurs when a severe depressive illness is accompanied by some form of psychosis, for example- break with reality, hallucinations, and delusions. A brief examination of these suffice-

When we talk about depression, what is subject of discourse is usually what healthcare providers called- Unipolar Major Depression (or major depressive disorder). To be diagnosed with unipolar major depression, a child or adolescent must have five or more of the following symptoms present most of the day for about two consecutive weeks.

Disruptive mood dysregulation disorder is more common than bipolar disorder particularly before adolescence, and symptoms tend to decrease as an adolescent moves into adulthood.

When in the depressed cycle, an individual can have any or all of the symptoms of a depressive disorder. When in the manic cycle, the individual may be overactive, overly talkative, and have a great deal of energy. Mania often affects thinking, judgment, and social behavior in ways that cause serious problems and embarrassment.

For bipolar disorders, it is not nearly as prevalent as other forms of depressive disorders and is characterized by mood changes, such as severe highs (mania) and lows (depression). Sometimes the mood switches are dramatic and rapid, but typically they are gradual.

Whereas Disruptive mood dysregulation disorder has an onset before the age of 10, and consists of chronic, severe, persistent irritability; children with this condition have frequent temper outbursts that include verbal rages and/or physical aggression, on the other hand, Premenstrual dysphoric disorder can occur at any time following the first occurrence of menstruation.

3.2 Understanding The Nexus Between Depression And Anxiety Among Children

Admittedly, children find it difficult to outgrow fears and worries without assistance. Intense fear for children is accompanied by symptoms like heart pounding, having trouble breathing, or feeling dizzy, shaky, or sweaty. Some of the signs and symptoms of anxiety and depression are shared with other conditions, such as trauma. Anxiety symptoms amongst children include trouble sleeping, as well as physical symptoms like fatigue, headaches, or stomachaches. These fears and worries interfere with a child's school, home, or play activities.

Children are more likely to develop anxiety and depression when they experience trauma or stress, when they are maltreated, when they are bullied or rejected As earlier discussed, depression could cause a child to make trouble or act unmotivated. Hence, it is wrong to outrightly label the child as a trouble-maker or lazy simply because many children have fears and worries making them sad from time to time. Although fears and worries are typical in children, persistent or extreme forms of fear and sadness feelings could be due to anxiety and depression.

Some anxiety disorders in children include:

- ➢ Fear of the future (general anxiety)
- ➢ Fear when away from parents/guardians (separation anxiety)

- ➤ Fear of crowed or going to places where they get to interact (social anxiety)
- ➤ Fear of things or situation, such as dogs, insects, or going to the doctor (phobias)

The first step to certainty in distinguishing mere anxiety from depression is to talk with a healthcare provider to get an evaluation upon noticing the symptoms of depression as herein set out. Consultation with a health provider can help determine if medication should be part of the treatment. Importantly, the American Academy of Child and Adolescent Psychiatry (AACAP) recommends that healthcare providers routinely screen children for behavioral and menta. health concerns.

The following pointers for helping children escape the cycle of anxiety have been identified:

-Encourage your child to talk about how he or she feels, but try not to ask leading questions

-Help the child to learn to tolerate anxiety and function well

-Do not promise a child that his or her fears are unrealistic, rather help the child plan as this can reduce the uncertainty in a healthy and effective way

-Encourage the child to engage in life and to let the anxiety take its natural course.

- Let the child have confidence that he or she is going to be okay despite the odds

- Help the child confront the things he or she is afraid of rather than avoid them

In addition to the above, the habits to inculcate in children battling depression are as follows:

-Participating in physical activities daily

-Getting the recommended amount of sleep each night based on age

-Eating a healthful diet centered on fruits, vegetables, seeds, whole grains, legumes, protein and nuts

-Practicing mindfulness or relaxation techniques

-Managing anxiety

3.3 Understanding The Nexus Between Depression And Comorbidity Among Children

When a person has two or more medical conditions, the conditions occurring together are called comorbidities. Depression can also increase the risk of other disorders setting in. The following comorbidities can compound the problems associated with depression and make the illness harder to treat, hence, children and adolescents being treated for depression should also be monitored for these issues:

- Anxiety disorders

- Attention deficit hyperactivity disorder

- Oppositional defiant disorder

- Substance use disorders

3.4 Warning Signs of Suicidal Behavior In Children

The following have been identified as signs that must be taken seriously in determining if a child or adolescent has suicidal tendencies:

-Talk of suicide, hopelessness, or helplessness

-Increased acting-out of undesirable behaviors

-Increased risk-taking behaviors

-Depressive symptoms (changes in eating, sleeping, activities)

-Social isolation, including isolation from the family

- Giving away possessions

-Frequent accidents

-Substance abuse

-Focus on morbid and negative themes

-Talk about death and dying

-Increased crying or reduced emotional expression

CHAPTER FOUR- APPRECIATING CHILDREN'S PSYCHOLOGICAL STATE

4.1 Appreciating Children's Emotional Development

Emotional development is variable among different children. The way children express emotions can be influenced by family and educators. The manner a child reacts to everyday routines, transitions, unfamiliar situations, and new people is influenced by his temperament. Temperament in this context refers to the traits that make a child unique, be it that the child is shy, exuberant, intense, or laid-back and it's a powerful factor in determining how he or she reacts to daily tasks. By the time they start school, children are more aware of their own feelings and the feelings of others. Thus, characteristics in a child's early years may turn into positive qualities as he or she grows. Temper tantrum could result where a child is angry due to the gap between the things the child wants to do and what he or she is actually able to do.

Whereas, feisty kids can be passionate and creative, slow-to-warm-up kids can be very thoughtful and sensitive. The differences when recognized leads to an appreciation which the child quickly recognizes, so parents must never feel demoralized with ways in which their child is very different from them. Each of these is present in every child—what differs is how they're expressed. For instance, as children develop, they begin to understand they can have more than one emotion when reacting to an event as long as they are similar.

In supporting emotional development, parents must pay attention to children's feelings and notice how they manage them. Hence, whatever your child's temperament, you must appreciate same and learn to honour those characteristics over other children's not minding that it is emotionally and physically exhausting. It is important for children to be understood for who they are since there is neither right nor wrong temperament. Children have different upbringing so tend to react differently; peculiar traits is what makes your child who he or she is. Some particular traits that parents should pay attention to in children are: intensity of reaction, activity level, tolerance for frustration, response to change, and reaction to new people.

4.2 Getting The Best Out Of Your Child

-Listening

-Interact regularly with your child

-Have some family moments when you hang out or simply spend time together indoors

-Get some favorite toys or books that aids learning

-Observe how your child reacts to new people and assist in putting restraints or building bonds

-Imbibe basic morals in your child

- Help your child to put feelings into words

-Teach your child to develop empathy for others

- Use familiar objects in teaching the child and use a dramatic voice while reading

-Do not label your child using negative words

- Praise your child when necessary and scold when necessary

-Aid in managing your child's emotion

- Help your child to understand the difference between his or her own and other people's feelings

- Listen to music, play, and pray together

-Emphasize the need for your child to separate feelings from behaviour

- Limit active play at least an hour before bedtime

-Be protective; remove your child from potentially explosive situations

- Offer advance notice on daily routines

-When your child is moody, understand what can brighten up the child

-Imbibe the spirit of persistence and perseverance in your child when faced with challenging tasks

- Join your child in his or her play

- Be firm when necessary

- Acknowledge your child's feelings and tune into your child's feelings

-Assist your child to think through solutions without doing the work yourself

-Lead by example

- Set limits on inappropriate expression of emotions

- Encourage problem-solving skills to manage emotions

-Give room for social interaction

- Give your child the chance to use his own resources and imagination

4.3 Regulating Your Children's Access to The Internet

It is vital for parents, educators and guardians to educate children and young people on risks and responsibilities they may encounter when using the Internet. The internet's reach extends beyond teens or children. Another reason for education on the internet and computer use is because you are better able to fully understand the dangers of them. Children and teens access the internet routinely and the nature of their internet experience has intensified. Numerous situations can develop online that have the potential to be dangerous. One of those situations is when personal information is exchanged with a stranger.

Equally, teens routinely use the internet for research and play, and view the medium as an extension of their real-world social environment by the use of e-mail, instant messaging, chat rooms, and web logs (blogging). Some reasons why internet use can be dangerous for children and teenagers are:

- Internet Predators

- False Identities

-Loss of privacy

- Having so many websites to choose from can be dangerous

-Cyber bullying

-Cyber stalking

 Flowing from the above, hereunder set out are guidelines for a safe internet experience:

-Parents and guardians are to know online friends just as they are expected to know other friends of their wards

-Personal information should be strictly kept private

-There should be guidelines for internet use, including the amount of time to stay online and sites that are off-limits

-Offline meeting should be with parents in attendance

-Inappropriate messages are to be treated with urgent attention

23

-Computers should be placed in open space for close monitoring

- It is important to have security updates, antivirus and anti-spyware software.

- Parental control software to block inappropriate websites and the use of teen/child-friendly browser is important

-Educate on online scams

- Equip teens and children with online literacy skills to responsibly reap the benefits Internet activity offers.

ABOUT THE AUTHOR

J. T. Mike is proficient in offering professional services and leads a top tier firm specializing in resolving various disorders. His instinctive aptitude for complex cases is unparallel and comes in handy in his writings which have enjoyed wide publication. His enthusiasm for resolving complex issues have distinguished him overtime and endeared him to clients across the globe. He is equally an astute bibliophile whose zeal for perfection routinely come into play whilst addressing variant disorders which factor in the peculiar needs of clients.